DIY Lotion Bars.
30 Amazing Lotion Bar Recipes

Table of content

Introduction

Lotion bars are extremely easy to make and extremely affordable. They don't require extensive equipment or knowledge and the great thing about them is that they will have you wondering why you ever bought regular lotion for years and years.

We spend hundreds of dollars every year buy lotions that are full of additives and chemicals that are terrible for our skin and horrible for our bodies. When we think we are doing something like moisturizing our skin, we are actually harming our bodies in other ways by introducing chemicals to our household.

By making your own lotion bars you can eliminate the chemicals and bring good wholesome things into your home.

Chapter 1 – Why Lotion Bars?

Let's first talk about what the big deal is about lotion bars and why they are beneficial to have in the first place. We'll also talk about some of the essential things you'll need if you're going to make your own lotion bars.

- **Safety** – We mentioned in the introduction about the fact that lotion you buy from the store is full of additives and chemicals you probably can't even pronounce. The great thing about these lotion bars is that the majority of them are full of ingredients that not only you know and are familiar with, but are so safe that you could eat.

That's not to say you would want to eat them, but generally speaking, if you have toddlers around you get the point. It's a nice comforting thought to know that most of these recipes are safe for the little ones in the house.

Note: Not all of the recipes are safe because some essential oils aren't safe for consumption as with a few other ingredients. However, the main ingredients in all the recipes (beeswax, the carrier oils, the butters, etc.) are all safe for consumption. If there is one you are unsure of you can check online or with the poison control center before making.

- **Moisturizing** – If you're worried about giving up regular lotion for a lotion bar, fear not. These lotion bars will give you just as much or even more moisture than you had with your traditional store bought lotion. You won't be disappointed with this department.

- **Make Great Gifts** – Lotion bars are excellent as party favors, baby shower gifts, Christmas gifts, teacher gifts, etc.; and the best part is how inexpensive they are to make. You can make a huge batch of them, find a cute mold and there you have Christmas gifts for everyone. Your friends and family will think you are talented and they don't know just how easy it is to accomplish the task.

- **Great for Pregnant Women** – Lotion bars are a wonderful gift for pregnant women because they can help with stretch marks and when made with the right essential oils it can provide a lot of relief during pregnancy.

  However, be careful, some essential oils are not safe for pregnant women and can induce labor – clary sage, for example – so make sure you know which are helpful and which aren't safe.

- **Get Yourself Some Fun Silicone Molds** – One of the things that you'll want to consider buying are some silicone molds to use for the lotion bars. You can always use muffin tins if you don't want to buy molds, but it is easier to have the molds if you are going to make lotion bars on a continual basis.

It's also fun to have the molds if you are going to use them for gifts and other things. They aren't essential to have, but you'll really enjoy having them in the long run.

Chapter 2 – First 10 Recipes

In this chapter are the first ten recipes for your lotion bars.

1) *Chocolate Peppermint Lotion Bars*

1/2 C Coconut Oil

½ C beeswax (grated)

1 C cocoa butter

½ C Shea butter

40 drops peppermint essential oil

1 T Vitamin E oil

Directions

Use a double boiler and mix together the following ingredients – coconut oil, beeswax, cocoa butter and Shea butter. Heat the double boiler to medium and stir everything together until everything mixes and melts together. Once everything is well combined, take it off the heat.

After you've removed it from the heat, let everything cool down for a couple minutes. Then stir in the essential oil drops and the vitamin E oil.

Once everything is mixed together pour the mixture into your mold. It will cool pretty quickly, so you'll want to be pretty fast getting it into the mold.

Note: You don't have to make this recipe with the essential oils. They aren't necessary, but they do add a little something extra to the smell.

Once they've cooled completely, pop them out of the molds and they are ready for immediate use.

2) Shea DIY Lotion Bar

½ C coconut oil

½ C Shea butter

½ C beeswax

½ t Vitamin E oil

Directions

Combine all ingredients except the Vitamin E oil in a double boiler and heat on medium heat until all ingredients melt and combine together. Stir constantly mixing together until everything is well combined.

After everything is mixed, bring it off the heat and let it cool for a minute, but not too long as it will harden. Then mix in the vitamin E oil. Immediately pour the mixture into your molds.

Once they are completely cooled, you can pop them out of the mold and use immediately.

3) Mango Butter DIY Lotion Bar

1/2 C coconut oil

½ C mango butter

½ C beeswax

½ t Vitamin E oil

Directions

Combine all ingredients except the Vitamin E oil in a double boiler and heat on medium heat until all ingredients melt and combine together. Stir constantly mixing together until everything is well combined.

After everything is mixed, bring it off the heat and let it cool for a minute, but not too long as it will harden. Then mix in the vitamin E oil. Immediately pour the mixture into your molds.

Once they are completely cooled, you can pop them out of the mold and use immediately.

4) Tri-Butter Lotion Bar

1 C coconut oil

1/3 C Shea butter

1/3 C cocoa butter

1/3 C mango butter

1 C beeswax

Directions

Combine all ingredients except the Vitamin E oil in a double boiler and heat on medium heat until all ingredients melt and combine together. Stir constantly mixing together until everything is well combined.

After everything is mixed, bring it off the heat and let it cool for a minute, but not too long as it will harden. Then mix in the vitamin E oil. Immediately pour the mixture into your molds.

Once they are completely cooled, you can pop them out of the mold and use immediately.

5) Lotion Bar Stick with Shea Butter

4 T Shea Butter

2 T coconut oil

4 t olive oil

4 t beeswax

30-40 drops of essential oils (your choice, see suggestions below)

Directions

Use a double boiler to melt all ingredients except the essential oils. Keep the heat on medium stirring constantly until everything is melted and the ingredients are well combined.

Take the mixture off the heat and slowly add the essential oils stirring them in gradually stirring gradually. Pour the mixture into your lotion bar tube and let it harden overnight. Then it is ready to use immediately.

Note: The lotion bar stick is kind of like a deodorant in that it is easier to apply than a regular lotion bar. It's mostly the storage that is different than the regular lotion bar. When using the essential oils consider using chamomile or orange to give it a nice scent but not something overpowering.

6) Lotion Bars for Pain Relief

2/3 C coconut oil

2/3 C Shea butter

2/3 C beeswax

2 T Menthol Crystals

20 drops Peppermint essential oil

1 t Arnica oil

Directions

In a double boiler, mix together the coconut oil, Shea butter and beeswax. Melt them together on medium heat stirring constantly until the ingredients mix together and are well combined.

After everything is mixed together, take the mixture off the heat and add in the menthol crystals. Once they have combined in with the mixture, add in the essential oils as well. After everything is well combined add the arnica oil. All of this should be done quickly because the mixture will start to cool making it difficult to stir the ingredient together.

Finally, pour the final mixture into the molds to set-up. After they have completely cooled, you can remove them from the mold.

7) Lotion Bar for Sensitive Skin

2/3 C beef tallow

2/3 C mango butter

4 T beeswax

30-40 drops essential oil (your choice)

Directions

Using a double boiler, combine all the ingredients together except the essential oils and melt them together over medium heat. Stir the ingredients constantly until they melt and they stir together smoothly.

Remove the mixture from the heat and stir in the essential oil you've chosen to add. Some essential oils aren't great for sensitive skin, so be cautious add them into the lotion bar at all. The essential oils are optional and if you choose to add them at all, keep it tame.

After you add essential oils (if adding), pour them into your molds and let them harden before popping them out of the molds and using them.

8) Bronzing Lotion Bar

1 C coffee infused coconut oil (see instructions below)

2/3 C beeswax

½ C Shea butter

2 T non-nano zinc oxide

1 t mineral makeup in dark color for more bronzing

Directions

First to infuse your coconut oil with coffee, take two cups of coconut oil and one cup of extremely finely ground coffee. Put them in a double boiler and cook them together over low heat stirring every few minutes. Leave it this way for a couple hours until the mixture takes on a dark color. Take it off the heat and let it cool just long enough to handle.

Then take the coffee infused oil and strain it through a cheesecloth (an old t-shirt also works), then let it cool. Then you're ready to go for the rest of the recipe.

To make the rest of the lotion bar, combine all ingredients in a double boiler and melt them all together over medium heat until the mixture is smooth.

Take it off medium heat and pour directly into your molds to harden. Wait over night or until the bars have completely cooled and harden before popping them out of the molds. They are ready for immediate use.

9) Lotion Bar to Help with Eczema

2/3 C Cocoa butter

6 T beeswax pastilles

½ C fermented cod liver oil (can be purchased online)

Essential oils (your choice)

Directions

Using a double boiler, melt the butter and the beeswax together over medium heat until both are well combined and smooth.

Once the mixture is smooth, remove it from the heat and let it cool just slightly and add the fermented cod liver oil and any essential oils you want to add. The essential oils are optional, but can add a wonderful aroma to your lotion bar.

After you've mixed in any essential oils and the fermented cod liver oil, quickly pour the mixture into your molds and let it cool the rest of the way. It should harden after six hours or over night. Then it will be ready to use.

10) DIY Vanilla Sunscreen Lotion Bar

½ C Coconut oil

½ C mango butter

½ C beeswax

1 T non-nano Zinc Oxide

½ t Vitamin E oil

Vanilla essential oil (a few drops should work, but you can add more if you think it needs it)

Directions

Using a double boiler, add the coconut oil, mango butter and beeswax into the boiler over medium heat. Mix the ingredients stirring frequently until they combine and are smooth.

Once they are mixed well, take them off the heat and add in the zinc oxide powder and your essential oil. Note: You can substitute a different essential oil here if you prefer a different scent. However, it is not recommended to use any citrus oil for the sunscreen bar as it will attract the sun and counteract the whole idea behind the bar.

Stir until both the powder and the oils are mixed in. Then pour into your molds and let the bars harden and solidify the rest of the day or over night.

Chapter 3 – Next Ten Recipes

Here are the recipes for the next ten lotion bars that you will find handy and helpful in your quest to make your own lotion bars.

11) DIY Bug-off Lotion Bar

½ C coconut oil

¼ C Shea butter

¼ C beeswax + 1 Tablespoon

1/8 C rosemary leaves (fresh or dried is fine)

½ t dried whole cloves

1 T thyme (dried or fresh is fine)

¼ t cinnamon

1/8 C dried catnip leaf

1 T mint leaf

½ t Vitamin E oil

Essential Oils (lavender and vanilla 10 drops of each)

Directions

Start by infusing the coconut oil with the herbs, so grab your double boiler and add the coconut oil and all the herbs – rosemary, cloves, thyme, cinnamon, catnip and mint. Leave this on a medium heat for around thirty minutes or until the coconut oil looks a darker shade and smells a lot like rosemary.

Then you'll need to strain out the herbs from the oil using a cheesecloth (an old t-shirt or small mesh strainer work too), and then place the infused oil back in the double boiler. Add in the Shea butter and the beeswax until they all melt together and become smooth.

Take off the heat and stir in the vitamin E oil and any essential oils you want to add. The essential oils are optional, but encourage just for the smell.

Pour into your molds and let set over night. After they have cooled and set completely they are ready for immediate use.

12) Simple Yet Lovely Lotion Bar

½ C beeswax (chopped)

½ C cocoa butter (chopped)

½ C coconut oil

2 T almond oil

2 T jojoba oil

Directions

For this lotion bar, try heating the beeswax and cocoa butter in the microwave. Only heat them for thirty seconds at a time, stirring in between each rotation. When they are finally melted all the way through and smooth when stirred, add the coconut oil, almond oil and jojoba oil. Stir to mix everything together.

Once everything is well combined, pour them into muffin tins with paper baking cups. You can wait for them to set and cool or even try putting them in refrigerator or freezer to speed up the process.

13) Green Tea Lotion Bar

½ C Food grade wax

1/3 C Mango butter

1/3 C Shea butter

¼ C Almond butter

1 T Green tea powder (Matcha)

1 T Coconut Oil

Directions

In a double boiler add the food grade wax, mango butter, almond butter, and coconut oil. Melt over medium heat until everything combines and is smooth.

After everything is smooth, remove from heat and stir in the green tea powder.

Immediately pour the mixture into the molds and then wait for them to finish cooling and setting up. Once they have completely cooled, they are ready for immediate use.

14) Oat Lotion Bar

½ C Food grade wax

1/3 C Cocoa butter

1/3 C Shea butter

¼ C Almond butter

1 T Oats

1 T Jojoba Oil

Directions

Use a food processor to pulse the oats until they are as fine as possible. Then get your double boiler and add the food grade wax, mango butter, almond butter, and jojoba oil. Melt over medium heat until everything combines and is smooth.

After everything is smooth, remove from heat and stir in the oat powder.

Immediately pour the mixture into the molds and then wait for them to finish cooling and setting up. Once they have completely cooled, they are ready for immediate use.

15) Lotion Bars with Lavender Essential Oil

1/3 C beeswax

1/3 C coconut oil

1/3 C cocoa butter

20 drops lavender essential oil

Directions

Combine all ingredients except the lavender oil in a double boiler and heat on medium heat until all ingredients melt and combine together. Stir constantly mixing together until everything is well combined.

After everything is mixed, bring it off the heat and let it cool for a minute, but not too long as it will harden. Then mix in the lavender oil. You can increase or decrease the amount of lavender oil depending on your personal preference. Immediately pour the mixture into your molds.

Once they are completely cooled, you can pop them out of the mold and use immediately.

16) Lotion Bar with Orange and Honey

3 T of Honey (raw is much better)

1 C beeswax

1 C Shea butter

2 T olive oil

10-12 drops orange essential oil

Directions

Combine the beeswax, Shea butter and coconut oil in a double boiler and heat on medium heat until all ingredients melt and combine together. Stir constantly mixing together until everything is well combined.

After everything is mixed, bring it off the heat and let it cool for a minute, but not too long as it will harden. Then mix in the olive oil, honey and orange essential oil. Immediately pour the mixture into your molds.

Once they are completely cooled, you can pop them out of the mold and use immediately.

17) Chocolate Orange Lotion Bar

1 ½ C coconut oil

1 ½ C beeswax (grated)

1 C cocoa butter

½ C Shea butter

40 drops orange essential oil

1 T vitamin E oil

Combine all ingredients except the Vitamin E and essential oils in a double boiler and heat on medium heat until all ingredients melt and combine together. Stir constantly mixing together until everything is well combined.

After everything is mixed, bring it off the heat and let it cool for a minute, but not too long as it will harden. Then mix in the vitamin E oil and orange essential oil. Immediately pour the mixture into your molds.

Once they are completely cooled, you can pop them out of the mold and use immediately.

18) The Basic DIY Lotion Bar

1 C Cocoa Butter

1 C Coconut Oil

1 C Beeswax (grated)

Combine all ingredients in a double boiler and heat on medium heat until all ingredients melt and combine together. Stir constantly mixing together until everything is well combined.

After everything is mixed, bring it off the heat, immediately pour the mixture into your molds.

Once they are completely cooled, you can pop them out of the mold and use immediately.

19) Lemon Lotion Bar

½ C beeswax

½ C Shea butter

½ C sweet almond oil

15-20 drops lemon essential oil

Directions

Combine all ingredients except the lemon essential oil in a double boiler and heat on medium heat until all ingredients melt and combine together. Stir constantly mixing together until everything is well combined.

After everything is mixed, bring it off the heat and let it cool for a minute, but not too long as it will harden. Then mix in the lemon oil. Immediately pour the mixture into your molds.

Once they are completely cooled, you can pop them out of the mold and use immediately.

20) Eucalyptus Lotion Bar

1 C Shea butter

1 C beeswax

1 C jojoba oil

15-20 drops Eucalyptus oil

Directions

Combine all ingredients except the essential oils in a double boiler and heat on medium heat until all ingredients melt and combine together. Stir constantly mixing together until everything is well combined.

After everything is mixed, bring it off the heat and let it cool for a minute, but not too long as it will harden. Then mix in the essential oil. Immediately pour the mixture into your molds.

Once they are completely cooled, you can pop them out of the mold and use immediately.

Chapter 4 – Last Ten Recipes

Here are the last ten lotion bar recipes to help you get started on your own journey to making lotion bars in your own life.

21) Rose Lotion Bar

1/2 C coconut oil

¼ C Shea butter

¾ C beeswax

A few drops of rose essential oil

Directions

Combine all ingredients except the rose oil in a double boiler and heat on medium heat until all ingredients melt and combine together. Stir constantly mixing together until everything is well combined.

After everything is mixed, bring it off the heat and let it cool for a minute, but not too long as it will harden. Then mix in the rose oil. You can add more rose oil as you see fit until you have the desired amount for your preference. Immediately pour the mixture into your molds.

Once they are completely cooled, you can pop them out of the mold and use immediately.

22) Orange and Geranium Lotion Bar

2 t honey

1/3 C beeswax

¼ C Shea butter

¼ C coconut oil

10 drops orange oil

5 drops geranium oil

Directions

Combine all ingredients except the essential oils and honey in a double boiler and heat on medium heat until all ingredients melt and combine together. Stir constantly mixing together until everything is well combined.

After everything is mixed, bring it off the heat and let it cool for a minute, but not too long as it will harden. Then mix in the essential oils and the honey. You can add more essential oils as you see fit until you have the desired amount for your preference. Immediately pour the mixture into your molds.

Once they are completely cooled, you can pop them out of the mold and use immediately.

23) *Café Latte Lotion Bar with a Hint of Mint*

1/3 C beeswax

¼ C cocoa butter

¼ C sweet almond oil

10 drops peppermint oil

5 T coffee beans

Combine all ingredients except the peppermint oil and coffee beans in a double boiler and heat on medium heat until all ingredients melt and combine together. Stir constantly mixing together until everything is well combined.

After everything is mixed, bring it off the heat and let it cool for a minute, but not too long as it will harden. Then mix in the peppermint oil. You can add more or less peppermint oil as you see fit until you have the desired amount for your preference. Immediately pour the mixture into your molds.

After you've poured them into the molds, top the bars with coffee beans and let them harden.

Once they are completely cooled, you can pop them out of the mold and use immediately.

24) Lavender and Honey Lotion Bar

4 T beeswax

¼ C coconut oil

2 T olive oil

2 t honey

8-10 drops Lavender essential oil

Directions

Combine all ingredients except the essential oil and the honey in a double boiler and heat on medium heat until all ingredients melt and combine together. Stir constantly mixing together until everything is well combined.

After everything is mixed, bring it off the heat and let it cool for a minute, but not too long as it will harden. Then mix in the essential oil and the honey. You can add more lavender oil as you see fit until you have the desired amount for your preference. Immediately pour the mixture into your molds.

Once they are completely cooled, you can pop them out of the mold and use immediately.

25) Lotion Bar with Calendula Essential Oil

4 T Shea butter

4 T beeswax (grated)

4 T calendula infused oil (can buy online)

Optional to add more essential oils

Directions

Combine all ingredients except any essential oils in a double boiler and heat on medium heat until all ingredients melt and combine together. Stir constantly mixing together until everything is well combined.

After everything is mixed, bring it off the heat and let it cool for a minute, but not too long as it will harden. Then mix in essential oils if adding. Immediately pour the mixture into your molds.

Once they are completely cooled, you can pop them out of the mold and use immediately.

26) Vanilla Face Lotion Bar

4 oz. coconut oil

1 oz. beeswax

½ t vanilla extract

Directions

Combine the coconut oil and beeswax in a double boiler and heat on medium heat until all ingredients melt and combine together. Stir constantly mixing together until everything is well combined.

After everything is mixed, bring it off the heat and let it cool for a minute, but not too long as it will harden. Then mix in the vanilla. You can add more vanilla as you see fit until you have the desired amount for your preference. Immediately pour the mixture into your molds.

Once they are completely cooled, you can pop them out of the mold and use immediately.

27) Calming Lotion Bar

½ C Shea butter

½ C cocoa butter

½ C beeswax

½ t vitamin E oil

15 drops Lavender essential oil

15 drops Neroli essential oil

10 drops Orange essential oil

Directions

Combine all ingredients except the essential oils and the vitamin E oil in a double boiler and heat on medium heat until all ingredients melt and combine together. Stir constantly mixing together until everything is well combined.

After everything is mixed, bring it off the heat and let it cool for a minute, but not too long as it will harden. Then mix in the vitamin E oil and the essential oils. You can add more essential oils as you see fit until you have the desired amount for your preference. Immediately pour the mixture into your molds or they will be too difficult to pour.

Once they are completely cooled, you can pop them out of the mold and use immediately.

28) Citrus Lotion Bar

½ C Shea butter

½ C cocoa butter

½ C beeswax

½ t vitamin E oil

15 drops Lime essential oil

15 drops Orange essential oil

10 drops Grapefruit essential oil

Directions

Combine all ingredients except the essential oils and the vitamin E oil in a double boiler and heat on medium heat until all ingredients melt and combine together. Stir constantly mixing together until everything is well combined.

After everything is mixed, bring it off the heat and let it cool for a minute, but not too long as it will harden. Then mix in the vitamin E oil and the essential oils. You can add more essential oils as you see fit until you have the desired amount for your preference. Immediately pour the mixture into your molds or they will be too difficult to pour.

Once they are completely cooled, you can pop them out of the mold and use immediately.

29) Flowering Lotion Bar

½ C Shea butter

½ C cocoa butter

½ C beeswax

½ t vitamin E oil

15 drops Jasmine essential oil

15 drops Ylang Ylang essential oil

10 drops Rose essential oil

Directions

Combine all ingredients except the essential oils and the vitamin E oil in a double boiler and heat on medium heat until all ingredients melt and combine together. Stir constantly mixing together until everything is well combined.

After everything is mixed, bring it off the heat and let it cool for a minute, but not too long as it will harden. Then mix in the vitamin E oil and the essential oils. You can add more essential oils as you see fit until you have the desired amount for your preference. Immediately pour the mixture into your molds or they will be too difficult to pour.

Once they are completely cooled, you can pop them out of the mold and use immediately.

30) Woodland Lotion Bar

½ C Shea butter

½ C cocoa butter

½ C beeswax

½ t vitamin E oil

15 drops Cedarwood essential oil

15 drops Lavender essential oil

10 drops Tea tree essential oil

Directions

Combine all ingredients except the essential oils and the vitamin E oil in a double boiler and heat on medium heat until all ingredients melt and combine together. Stir constantly mixing together until everything is well combined.

After everything is mixed, bring it off the heat and let it cool for a minute, but not too long as it will harden. Then mix in the vitamin E oil and the essential oils. You can add more essential oils as you see fit until you have the desired amount for your preference. Immediately pour the mixture into your molds or they will be too difficult to pour.

Once they are completely cooled, you can pop them out of the mold and use immediately.

Conclusion

It's really a lot of fun making your own lotion bars. As you can see from the recipes, they aren't a lot of work to make and they aren't very expensive. You'll enjoy having them around the house – in the bathroom, the kitchen and even keeping one with you as you go about your daily activities.

You won't regret making the switch from regular lotion bought in the store to making your own lotion. You can find the scents and flavors that you enjoy best rather than be stuck opening and smelling all the different bottles in the store or buying something and hoping that it smells good once you get home.

Instead you can make something at home and know from the moment you make it that it's going to smell good, moisturize your skin and leave you feeling good all day long.

FREE Bonus Reminder

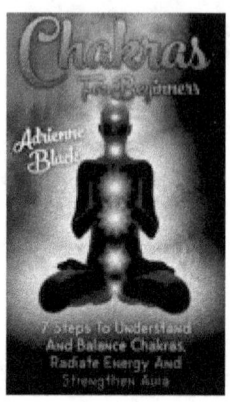

If you have not grabbed it yet, please go ahead and download your special bonus E book *"Chakras for Beginners. 7 Steps To Understand And Balance Chakras, Radiate Energy, And Strengthen Aura".*

Simply Click the Button Below

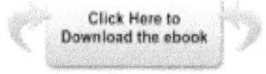

OR Go to This Page

http://lifehacksworld.com/free

BONUS #2: More Free & Discounted Books & Products

Do you want to receive more Free/Discounted Books or Products?

We have a mailing list where we send out our new Books or Products when they go free or with a discount on Amazon. Click on the link below to sign up for Free & Discount Book & Product Promotions.

=> Sign Up for Free & Discount Book & Product Promotions <=

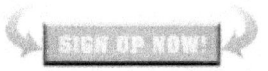

OR Go to this URL

http://zbit.ly/1WBb1Ek